This publication is intended to provide educational information for the reader on the covered subjects. It is not intended to take the place of personalized medical counseling, diagnosis, and treatment from a trained healthcare professional.

ISBN 978-1-998455-49-2 (Paperback)
ISBN 978-1-998455-50-8 (eBook)

Printed and bound in USA
Published by Loons Press

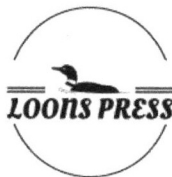

LOONS PRESS

I0096767

Table Of Contents

How To Prevent Stomach Cancer

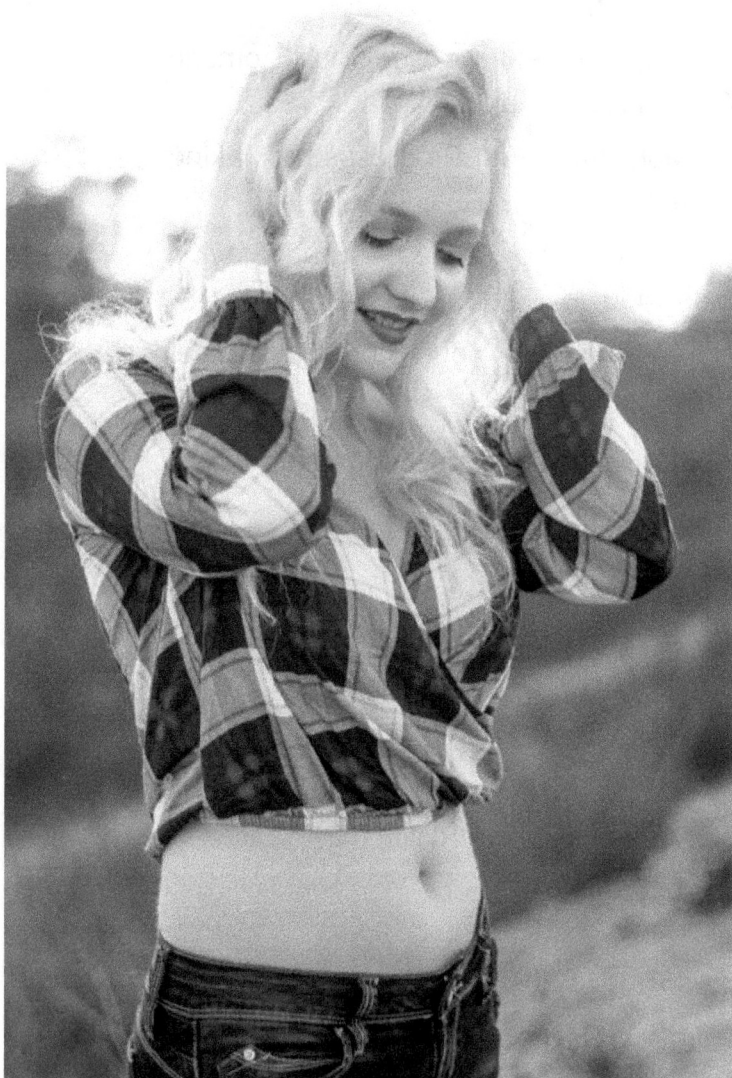

Strategies for Reducing Your Risk

Another common risk factor for stomach cancer is infection with the bacterium Helicobacter pylori (H. pylori). This bacterium is known to cause inflammation of the stomach lining, which can increase the risk of developing stomach cancer. If you have been diagnosed with an H. pylori infection, it is important to seek treatment from a healthcare professional to reduce your risk of developing stomach cancer.

Smoking and heavy alcohol consumption are also significant risk factors for stomach cancer. Both of these habits can damage the cells in the stomach lining and increase the risk of developing cancerous cells. If you smoke or drink heavily, it is important to take steps to quit or reduce your consumption to lower your risk of developing stomach cancer.

Family history of stomach cancer is another important risk factor to consider. If you have a close relative who has been diagnosed with stomach cancer, your risk of developing the disease may be higher. It is important to talk to your healthcare provider about your family history and any concerns you may have about your risk of developing stomach cancer.

This book aims to provide individuals at risk of stomach cancer with the knowledge and tools they need to protect their health and well-being.

Common Risk Factors for Stomach Cancer

Stomach cancer is a serious and potentially life-threatening disease that affects millions of people worldwide each year. While the exact causes of stomach cancer are not fully understood, there are several common risk factors that have been identified. By understanding these risk factors and taking steps to address them, you can significantly reduce your risk of developing stomach cancer.

One of the most well-known risk factors for stomach cancer is a diet high in salt and processed foods. Consuming too much salt can damage the lining of the stomach and increase the risk of developing cancerous cells. To reduce your risk, it is important to limit your intake of salty and processed foods and opt for a diet rich in fruits, vegetables, and whole grains.

Prevention strategies for stomach cancer include maintaining a healthy diet that is high in fruits, vegetables, and whole grains, and low in processed and fatty foods. It is also important to avoid smoking and limit alcohol consumption, as these habits have been linked to an increased risk of stomach cancer. Regular exercise and maintaining a healthy weight can also help reduce the risk of developing stomach cancer.

Regular screenings and check-ups with a healthcare provider are essential for early detection and treatment of stomach cancer. Symptoms of stomach cancer can include unexplained weight loss, persistent indigestion, abdominal pain, and bloating. If you experience any of these symptoms, it is important to seek medical attention promptly to rule out the possibility of stomach cancer.

By understanding the risk factors and prevention strategies for stomach cancer, individuals can take proactive steps to reduce their risk of developing this deadly disease. With early detection and treatment, the chances of successfully overcoming stomach cancer are greatly improved.

Chapter 1

Understanding Stomach Cancer Risk Factors

Introduction to Stomach Cancer

Stomach cancer, also known as gastric cancer, is a serious and potentially life-threatening disease that affects the lining of the stomach. This type of cancer is particularly dangerous because it often goes undetected until it reaches advanced stages, making it more difficult to treat. Understanding the risk factors and prevention strategies for stomach cancer is crucial for individuals who may be at risk.

One of the key risk factors for stomach cancer is age, with the disease being more common in older individuals. Other risk factors include a family history of stomach cancer, a diet high in salty and smoked foods, chronic gastritis, and infection with the Helicobacter pylori bacteria. Individuals with these risk factors should be particularly vigilant about monitoring their health and taking steps to reduce their risk of developing stomach cancer.

In conclusion, there are several common risk factors for stomach cancer that can significantly increase your risk of developing the disease. By taking steps to address these risk factors, such as improving your diet, seeking treatment for H. pylori infection, quitting smoking and reducing alcohol consumption, and discussing your family history with your healthcare provider, you can greatly reduce your risk of developing stomach cancer. Remember, prevention is key when it comes to reducing your risk of developing this serious disease.

Genetic Factors and Stomach Cancer

When it comes to preventing stomach cancer, it's important to understand the role that genetic factors can play in increasing your risk. While lifestyle choices such as diet and exercise certainly play a significant role in your overall risk for developing stomach cancer, genetics can also play a role in determining your susceptibility to this disease. By understanding how genetic factors can influence your risk, you can take proactive steps to reduce your chances of developing stomach cancer.

One of the most well-known genetic factors associated with stomach cancer is a family history of the disease. If you have a close family member, such as a parent or sibling, who has been diagnosed with stomach cancer, your own risk for developing the disease is significantly higher. This is because certain genetic mutations can be passed down from generation to generation, increasing the likelihood that you may inherit a predisposition to stomach cancer. If you have a family history of stomach cancer, it's important to speak with your healthcare provider about genetic testing and other preventive measures you can take to reduce your risk.

In addition to family history, certain genetic mutations have been linked to an increased risk of developing stomach cancer. For example, mutations in the CDH1 gene have been associated with a condition known as hereditary diffuse gastric cancer (HDGC), which greatly increases the risk of developing stomach cancer at a young age. If you have a known genetic mutation that predisposes you to stomach cancer, it's important to work closely with your healthcare provider to develop a personalized prevention plan that takes into account your genetic risk factors.

While genetic factors can certainly play a role in increasing your risk for stomach cancer, it's important to remember that they are just one piece of the puzzle. Lifestyle factors such as smoking, a diet high in salt and processed foods, and being overweight are also significant risk factors for stomach cancer. By addressing these modifiable risk factors in addition to any genetic predispositions you may have, you can greatly reduce your overall risk for developing stomach cancer. Remember, knowledge is power when it comes to preventing stomach cancer, so be sure to stay informed about both your genetic risk factors and the lifestyle choices you can make to protect your health.

In conclusion, genetic factors can play a significant role in determining your risk for developing stomach cancer. If you have a family history of the disease or known genetic mutations that increase your risk, it's important to work closely with your healthcare provider to develop a personalized prevention plan. By addressing both genetic and lifestyle factors that can influence your risk for stomach cancer, you can take proactive steps to protect your health and reduce your chances of developing this disease.

Remember, prevention is key when it comes to stomach cancer, so be sure to prioritize your health and well-being by staying informed and taking action to reduce your risk.

Lifestyle Factors That Increase Stomach Cancer Risk

Stomach cancer is a serious and potentially life-threatening disease that affects millions of people worldwide each year. While there are many factors that can contribute to an individual's risk of developing stomach cancer, certain lifestyle factors have been shown to significantly increase the likelihood of developing this disease.

By understanding these lifestyle factors and making changes to reduce your risk, you can take proactive steps to protect your health and lower your chances of developing stomach cancer.

How To Prevent Stomach Cancer

One lifestyle factor that can increase the risk of stomach cancer is a poor diet high in processed and red meats, as well as foods that are high in salt and preservatives. Consuming a diet that is rich in fruits, vegetables, whole grains, and lean proteins can help to reduce your risk of developing stomach cancer.

By making healthier food choices and incorporating more plant-based foods into your diet, you can lower your risk of developing this disease.

Another lifestyle factor that can increase the risk of stomach cancer is smoking. Tobacco smoke contains harmful chemicals that can damage the lining of the stomach and increase the likelihood of developing cancerous cells.

By quitting smoking and avoiding exposure to secondhand smoke, you can significantly reduce your risk of developing stomach cancer. If you need help quitting smoking, there are resources available to support you in this important lifestyle change.

In addition to diet and smoking, excessive alcohol consumption has also been linked to an increased risk of stomach cancer. Alcohol can irritate the lining of the stomach and increase inflammation, which can contribute to the development of cancerous cells.

By reducing your alcohol intake and drinking in moderation, you can help to lower your risk of stomach cancer. Choosing non-alcoholic beverages or limiting your alcohol consumption to special occasions can be effective strategies for reducing your risk.

Lastly, another lifestyle factor that can increase the risk of stomach cancer is obesity. Being overweight or obese can increase inflammation in the body and contribute to the development of cancerous cells. By maintaining a healthy weight through regular exercise and a balanced diet, you can help to reduce your risk of developing stomach cancer.

Incorporating physical activity into your daily routine, such as walking, jogging, or swimming, can help you achieve and maintain a healthy weight and lower your risk of stomach cancer. By addressing these lifestyle factors and making positive changes, you can take control of your health and reduce your risk of developing stomach cancer.

How To Prevent Stomach Cancer

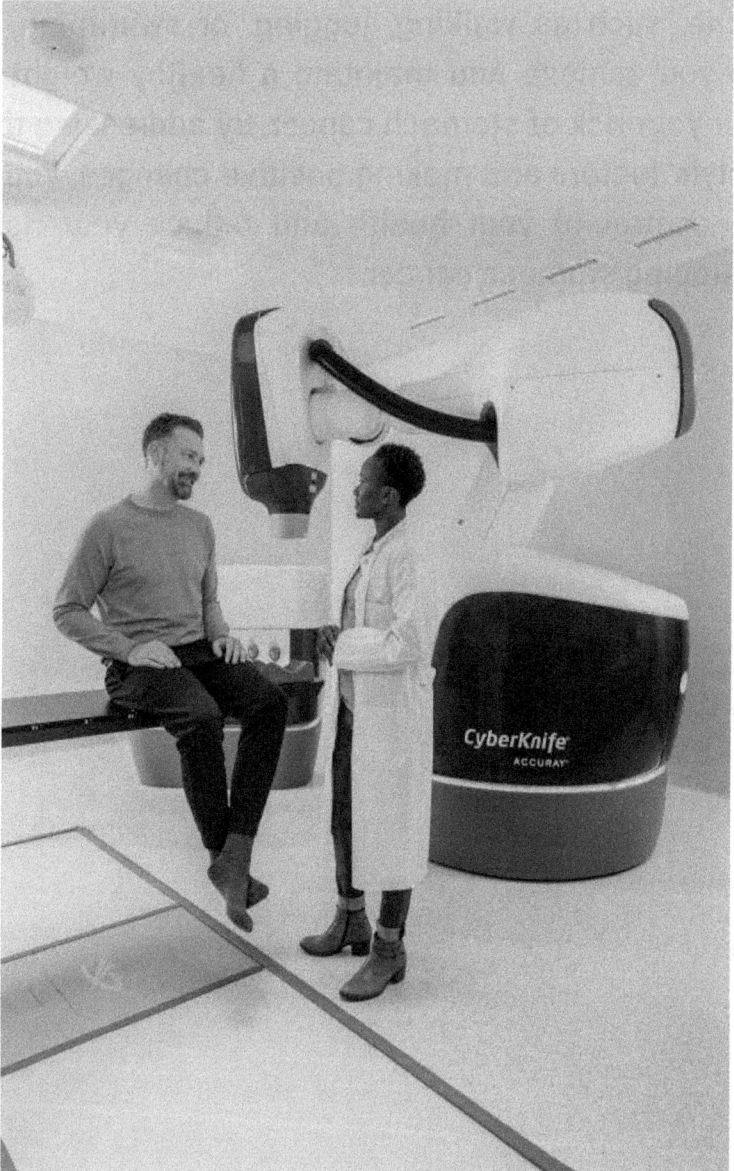

Strategies for Reducing Your Risk

Chapter 2

Screening and Early Detection

Importance of Early Detection in Stomach Cancer

Stomach cancer is a serious and potentially life-threatening disease that affects millions of people each year. One of the most important factors in successfully treating stomach cancer is early detection. The earlier stomach cancer is detected, the more likely it is that treatment will be effective. This is why it is crucial for individuals who have a high risk of developing stomach cancer to be vigilant about monitoring their health and seeking medical attention if they experience any symptoms.

Early detection of stomach cancer can greatly increase a patient's chances of survival. When stomach cancer is caught in its early stages, before it has had a chance to spread to other parts of the body, it is much more likely to be successfully treated.

This is why regular screenings and check-ups are so important for individuals who are at risk of developing stomach cancer. By detecting stomach cancer early, doctors can develop a treatment plan that is tailored to the individual patient's needs, increasing the chances of a positive outcome.

In addition to increasing the chances of successful treatment, early detection of stomach cancer can also help to reduce the overall impact of the disease on a patient's quality of life. Stomach cancer can cause a range of symptoms, including abdominal pain, nausea, and weight loss. By catching stomach cancer early, doctors can work to manage these symptoms and help patients maintain a better quality of life throughout their treatment journey.

For individuals who have a high risk of developing stomach cancer, it is important to be proactive about monitoring their health and seeking medical attention if they notice any concerning symptoms. This may involve regular screenings, such as endoscopies or imaging tests, as well as maintaining a healthy lifestyle and following a nutritious diet.

By taking these steps, individuals can help to increase their chances of early detection and successful treatment if they are diagnosed with stomach cancer.

In conclusion, early detection is crucial in the fight against stomach cancer. By being proactive about monitoring their health and seeking medical attention if they notice any concerning symptoms, individuals who are at risk of developing stomach cancer can greatly increase their chances of successful treatment and a better quality of life. Remember, early detection saves lives.

Screening Methods for Stomach Cancer

Stomach cancer is a serious and potentially life-threatening disease that affects millions of people worldwide. Fortunately, there are several screening methods available that can help detect stomach cancer in its early stages when it is most treatable.

In this chapter, we will discuss some of the most common screening methods for stomach cancer and how they can help reduce your risk of developing this deadly disease.

One of the most common screening methods for stomach cancer is an upper endoscopy, also known as a gastroscopy. During this procedure, a thin, flexible tube with a camera on the end is passed through the mouth and into the stomach. This allows the doctor to visually inspect the lining of the stomach for any abnormalities or signs of cancer. If any suspicious areas are found, a biopsy can be taken and sent to a lab for further testing.

Another screening method for stomach cancer is a barium swallow test, also known as an upper GI series. During this test, the patient drinks a chalky liquid containing barium, which coats the lining of the stomach and makes it easier to see on X-rays. The doctor can then take X-rays of the stomach to look for any abnormalities or signs of cancer. While this test is not as effective as an endoscopy for detecting stomach cancer, it can still be useful in certain situations.

In addition to these screening methods, there are also blood tests available that can help detect stomach cancer. One such test is the CA 19-9 test, which measures the levels of a specific protein in the blood that can be elevated in patients with stomach cancer.

While this test is not specific to stomach cancer and can be elevated in other conditions, it can still be a useful tool in conjunction with other screening methods.

It is important for people who are at risk of stomach cancer to talk to their doctor about which screening methods may be appropriate for them. By undergoing regular screenings, individuals can increase their chances of detecting stomach cancer in its early stages when it is most treatable.

Remember, early detection is key to successfully treating stomach cancer and improving your chances of survival. Take charge of your health and reduce your risk of stomach cancer by staying informed and proactive about screening methods.

Understanding Biopsies and Other Diagnostic Tests

If you have been identified as someone who is at risk for stomach cancer, it is important to understand the various diagnostic tests that can help detect the disease early on. One common test used to diagnose stomach cancer is a biopsy, where a small sample of tissue is taken from the stomach lining and examined under a microscope for the presence of cancer cells. Biopsies are often performed during an endoscopy, where a thin, flexible tube with a camera is inserted into the stomach to allow doctors to see the interior of the stomach and take tissue samples.

In addition to biopsies, there are other diagnostic tests that can help detect stomach cancer, such as imaging tests like CT scans, MRIs, and PET scans. These tests can help doctors see if there are any abnormalities in the stomach that may indicate the presence of cancer. Blood tests may also be used to look for certain markers that are associated with stomach cancer, although these tests are not always definitive on their own.

How To Prevent Stomach Cancer

It is important to work closely with your healthcare provider to determine which diagnostic tests are appropriate for you based on your individual risk factors and symptoms. Regular screenings and tests can help detect stomach cancer in its early stages when it is more treatable.

If you have a family history of stomach cancer or other risk factors, your doctor may recommend more frequent screenings to help catch any potential issues early on.

Understanding the various diagnostic tests available for stomach cancer can help you take control of your health and reduce your risk of developing the disease. By staying proactive and working closely with your healthcare provider, you can catch any potential issues early on and take steps to prevent stomach cancer from developing.

Remember, early detection is key in successfully treating stomach cancer, so don't hesitate to ask your doctor about which tests are right for you.

What to Expect During a Stomach Cancer Screening

Stomach cancer is a serious disease that can be difficult to detect in its early stages. However, there are screening tests available that can help identify the presence of stomach cancer before symptoms develop.

If you have risk factors for stomach cancer, it is important to be aware of what to expect during a stomach cancer screening.

One common screening test for stomach cancer is an upper endoscopy, also known as a gastroscopy. During this procedure, a thin, flexible tube with a camera on the end is inserted through the mouth and into the stomach.

This allows the doctor to examine the lining of the stomach for any abnormalities or signs of cancer. The procedure is typically done under sedation to make it more comfortable for the patient.

Another screening test for stomach cancer is an upper gastrointestinal series, also known as a barium swallow. During this test, the patient drinks a liquid containing barium, which coats the stomach and makes it visible on X-rays. The X-rays can then be used to look for any abnormalities in the stomach lining that may indicate the presence of cancer.

In some cases, a biopsy may be taken during an endoscopy or other procedure to confirm a diagnosis of stomach cancer. This involves removing a small sample of tissue from the stomach lining and examining it under a microscope for signs of cancer cells. While a biopsy can be uncomfortable, it is an important step in accurately diagnosing stomach cancer.

It is important to discuss the results of your screening tests with your doctor to determine the next steps in your care. If stomach cancer is detected, your doctor will work with you to develop a treatment plan that is tailored to your specific needs. Early detection of stomach cancer can greatly improve the chances of successful treatment and recovery.

Overall, knowing what to expect during a stomach cancer screening can help ease any anxiety or concerns you may have about the process. By staying informed and proactive about your health, you can take steps to reduce your risk of stomach cancer and increase the likelihood of early detection and successful treatment.

How To Prevent Stomach Cancer

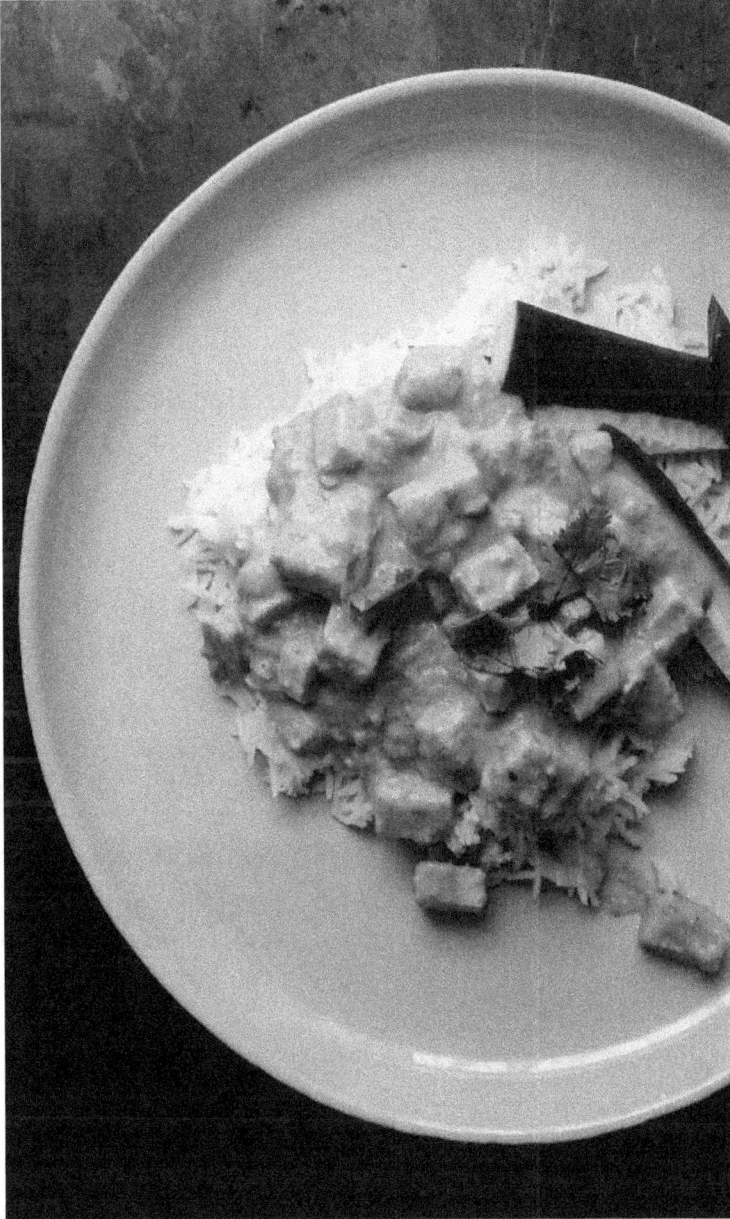

Strategies for Reducing Your Risk

Chapter 3

Dietary Strategies for Stomach Cancer Prevention

The Role of Diet in Stomach Cancer Prevention

Diet plays a crucial role in preventing stomach cancer, especially for those who are at risk due to genetic factors or lifestyle choices. By making conscious decisions about what you eat, you can significantly reduce your risk of developing this deadly disease. In this subchapter, we will explore the impact of diet on stomach cancer prevention and provide practical tips for incorporating healthy eating habits into your daily routine.

One of the most important factors in preventing stomach cancer through diet is the consumption of fruits and vegetables. These foods are rich in antioxidants, vitamins, and minerals that help protect the cells in your stomach from damage and reduce inflammation.

Aim to include a variety of colorful fruits and vegetables in your diet, such as leafy greens, berries, citrus fruits, and cruciferous vegetables like broccoli and cauliflower.

Another key component of a stomach cancer prevention diet is whole grains. Foods like whole wheat bread, brown rice, quinoa, and oats are high in fiber, which helps regulate digestion and promote a healthy gut microbiome. A healthy gut is essential for preventing stomach cancer, as it plays a crucial role in the immune system and the body's ability to fight off cancerous cells.

In addition to fruits, vegetables, and whole grains, it is important to limit your intake of processed and red meats. These foods have been linked to an increased risk of stomach cancer, likely due to their high levels of saturated fats and additives. Instead, opt for lean proteins like fish, poultry, beans, and tofu. These sources of protein are not only healthier for your stomach but also provide essential nutrients for overall health and well-being.

In conclusion, a diet rich in fruits, vegetables, whole grains, and lean proteins can significantly reduce your risk of developing stomach cancer. By making small changes to your eating habits and incorporating these healthy foods into your daily routine, you can take proactive steps towards preventing this deadly disease. Remember, prevention is always better than cure, so start making smart choices about what you eat today to protect your stomach health for years to come.

Foods to Include in a Stomach Cancer Prevention Diet

Stomach cancer is a serious disease that can have a significant impact on your health and well-being. However, there are steps you can take to reduce your risk of developing this condition. One of the most important ways to prevent stomach cancer is to follow a healthy diet that includes plenty of fruits, vegetables, and whole grains. In this subchapter, we will discuss some of the foods that you should include in your stomach cancer prevention diet.

One of the key components of a stomach cancer prevention diet is fruits and vegetables. These foods are rich in vitamins, minerals, and antioxidants that can help protect your stomach cells from damage that may lead to cancer. Aim to include a variety of colorful fruits and vegetables in your diet, such as berries, citrus fruits, leafy greens, and cruciferous vegetables like broccoli and cauliflower.

Whole grains are another important part of a stomach cancer prevention diet. Foods like brown rice, whole wheat bread, and quinoa are high in fiber, which can help keep your digestive system healthy and may reduce your risk of developing stomach cancer. Additionally, whole grains are a good source of vitamins and minerals that are essential for overall health.

Lean protein sources, such as chicken, fish, and tofu, should also be included in a stomach cancer prevention diet. These foods provide essential nutrients that support a strong immune system and help maintain healthy stomach tissue.

Aim to include a variety of protein sources in your diet to ensure you are getting all the nutrients you need to support your overall health and reduce your risk of developing stomach cancer.

In addition to these foods, it is important to limit your intake of processed meats, red meats, and foods that are high in salt and unhealthy fats. These foods have been linked to an increased risk of stomach cancer and should be consumed in moderation. Instead, focus on including a variety of nutrient-dense foods in your diet that can help support your overall health and reduce your risk of developing stomach cancer.

By following a stomach cancer prevention diet that includes plenty of fruits, vegetables, whole grains, and lean proteins, you can help reduce your risk of developing this serious disease. Remember to also maintain a healthy weight, exercise regularly, and avoid smoking and excessive alcohol consumption to further reduce your risk. Making these lifestyle changes can have a significant impact on your overall health and well-being, and may help lower your risk of developing stomach cancer.

Foods to Avoid to Reduce Stomach Cancer Risk

Stomach cancer is a serious disease that can be influenced by dietary choices. In this subchapter, we will discuss the foods that should be avoided in order to reduce your risk of stomach cancer. By making informed decisions about what you eat, you can take steps towards preventing this deadly illness.

One of the key foods to avoid in order to reduce your risk of stomach cancer is processed meats. These meats are often high in nitrates and nitrites, which have been linked to an increased risk of stomach cancer. Instead, opt for fresh, lean meats that are cooked at home and free from added preservatives.

Another food that should be avoided is pickled and salted foods. These foods are often high in sodium, which can irritate the lining of the stomach and increase the risk of developing stomach cancer. Instead, choose fresh fruits and vegetables as snacks or incorporate them into your meals to reduce your intake of pickled and salted foods.

Highly processed and fried foods should also be limited in order to reduce your risk of stomach cancer. These foods are often high in trans fats, which have been linked to an increased risk of developing various types of cancer, including stomach cancer. Instead, focus on incorporating whole grains, lean proteins, and healthy fats into your diet to reduce your risk.

Alcohol and tobacco use should also be avoided in order to reduce your risk of stomach cancer. Both alcohol and tobacco have been linked to an increased risk of developing stomach cancer, so it is important to avoid these substances altogether. Instead, opt for non-alcoholic beverages and seek support to quit smoking in order to reduce your risk.

By making informed choices about the foods you eat and avoiding those that are linked to an increased risk of stomach cancer, you can take steps towards reducing your overall risk of developing this deadly disease. Remember to consult with a healthcare provider or nutritionist for personalized recommendations tailored to your specific risk factors and health needs.

Tips for Healthy Eating to Lower Stomach Cancer Risk

Stomach cancer is a serious and potentially life-threatening disease that can be influenced by various factors, including diet. For those at risk of developing stomach cancer, making healthy food choices is essential in lowering their risk.

In this subchapter, we will discuss some tips for healthy eating that can help reduce the risk of stomach cancer and promote overall well-being.

One important tip for lowering the risk of stomach cancer through diet is to incorporate a variety of fruits and vegetables into your meals. Fruits and vegetables are rich in vitamins, minerals, and antioxidants that can help protect the stomach lining from damage and inflammation.

Aim to include a rainbow of colors in your diet, as each color represents different nutrients that can benefit your health.

Another key tip is to limit the consumption of processed and red meats. Studies have shown that a high intake of processed and red meats is associated with an increased risk of stomach cancer. Instead, opt for lean proteins such as fish, poultry, beans, and nuts. These sources of protein are not only healthier for the stomach but also provide essential nutrients for overall health.

In addition to choosing healthy foods, it is important to pay attention to portion sizes and meal timing. Eating large meals and snacking late at night can put unnecessary strain on the stomach and increase the risk of stomach cancer. Try to eat smaller, more frequent meals throughout the day and avoid eating right before bedtime to give your stomach a chance to digest properly.

Lastly, staying hydrated is crucial for maintaining a healthy digestive system and reducing the risk of stomach cancer. Drinking plenty of water throughout the day helps to keep the stomach lining healthy and aids in digestion.

Limiting the consumption of sugary beverages and alcohol is also important, as these can irritate the stomach lining and increase the risk of cancer.

By following these tips for healthy eating, individuals at risk of stomach cancer can take proactive steps to lower their risk and improve their overall health and well-being.

How To Prevent Stomach Cancer

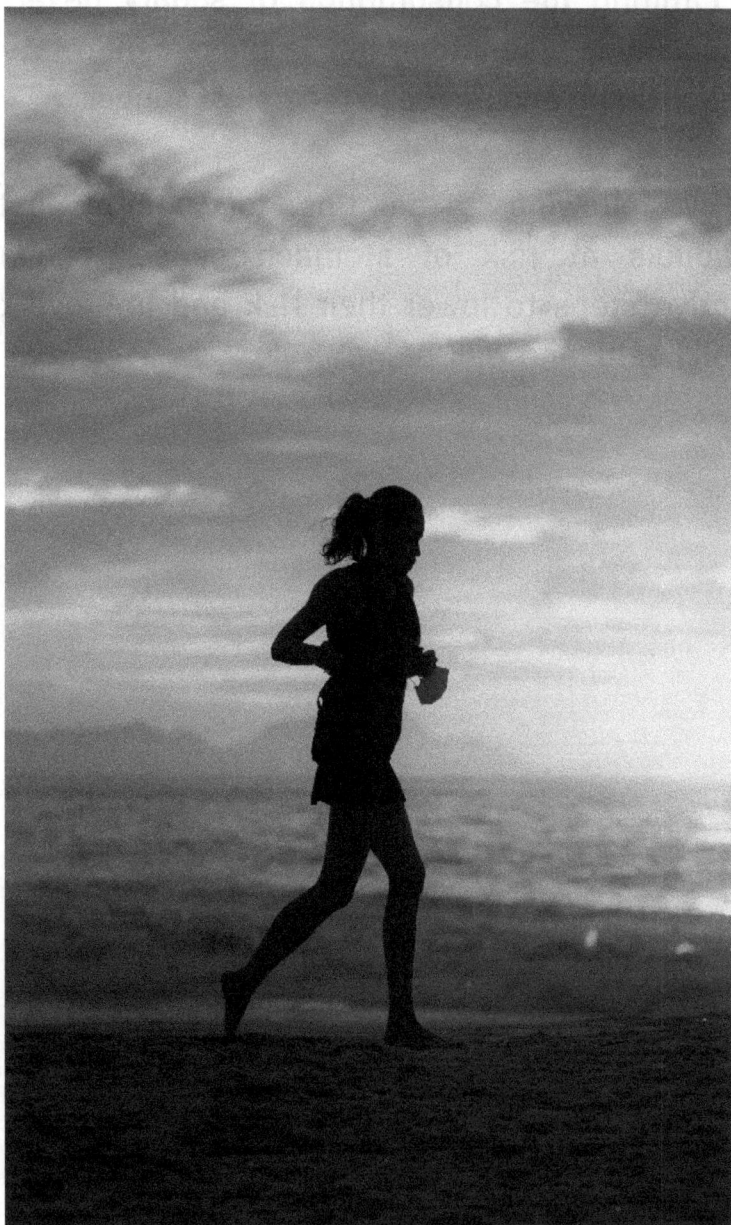

Strategies for Reducing Your Risk

Chapter 4

Lifestyle Changes for Stomach Cancer Prevention

The Impact of Lifestyle Choices on Stomach Cancer Risk

Stomach cancer is a serious disease that can have a significant impact on your health and well-being. One of the key factors that can influence your risk of developing stomach cancer is your lifestyle choices. By making informed decisions about your diet, exercise, and other habits, you can help reduce your risk of this potentially deadly disease.

Diet plays a crucial role in determining your risk of stomach cancer. Consuming a diet high in salty, smoked, or pickled foods can increase your risk, while eating plenty of fruits, vegetables, and whole grains can help lower it. It's also important to limit your intake of processed meats and red meats, as these have been linked to an increased risk of stomach cancer. By making healthy choices about the foods you eat, you can help protect yourself from this disease.

Regular exercise is another important factor in reducing your risk of stomach cancer. Studies have shown that people who are physically active have a lower risk of developing this type of cancer than those who are sedentary.

Aim for at least 30 minutes of moderate exercise most days of the week to help protect yourself from stomach cancer. Not only will exercise help reduce your risk of cancer, but it can also improve your overall health and well-being.

In addition to diet and exercise, other lifestyle choices can impact your risk of stomach cancer. For example, smoking and excessive alcohol consumption have both been linked to an increased risk of this disease.

If you smoke, quitting can help lower your risk of stomach cancer, as well as many other serious health conditions. Similarly, limiting your alcohol intake to no more than one drink per day for women or two drinks per day for men can help protect you from stomach cancer.

Overall, making healthy lifestyle choices can have a significant impact on your risk of developing stomach cancer. By eating a balanced diet, exercising regularly, avoiding tobacco and excessive alcohol consumption, and maintaining a healthy weight, you can help reduce your risk of this disease.

By following these guidelines and working with your healthcare provider to monitor your health, you can take proactive steps to protect yourself from stomach cancer and live a healthier, happier life.

Smoking and Alcohol Consumption in Relation to Stomach Cancer

Smoking and alcohol consumption are two major risk factors that have been linked to the development of stomach cancer. In this subchapter, we will explore the relationship between these habits and the increased risk of stomach cancer. It is important for individuals who are at risk of stomach cancer to understand how these lifestyle choices can impact their overall health and well-being.

Research has shown that smoking is associated with an increased risk of developing stomach cancer. The chemicals found in tobacco smoke can damage the lining of the stomach, leading to inflammation and an increased risk of cancerous growths.

Individuals who smoke are more likely to develop stomach cancer compared to non-smokers. To reduce your risk of stomach cancer, it is important to quit smoking and avoid exposure to secondhand smoke.

Similarly, alcohol consumption has been linked to an increased risk of stomach cancer. Heavy alcohol consumption can irritate the lining of the stomach and increase the production of stomach acid, which can contribute to the development of cancerous cells.

Individuals who regularly consume alcohol are at a higher risk of developing stomach cancer compared to those who drink in moderation or abstain from alcohol altogether. To reduce your risk of stomach cancer, it is important to limit your alcohol intake and seek help if you are struggling with alcohol addiction.

In addition to quitting smoking and limiting alcohol consumption, there are other lifestyle changes that can help reduce your risk of developing stomach cancer. Eating a healthy diet rich in fruits, vegetables, and whole grains can help protect against stomach cancer. Maintaining a healthy weight, staying physically active, and avoiding processed and preserved foods can also help lower your risk. By making these changes to your lifestyle, you can take proactive steps to reduce your risk of stomach cancer and improve your overall health and well-being.

In conclusion, smoking and alcohol consumption are two major risk factors that have been linked to an increased risk of developing stomach cancer. By understanding the relationship between these habits and stomach cancer, individuals who are at risk can take steps to reduce their risk and improve their overall health. Quitting smoking, limiting alcohol consumption, eating a healthy diet, and staying physically active are all important strategies for preventing stomach cancer. By making these lifestyle changes, you can reduce your risk of developing stomach cancer and live a healthier, happier life.

Exercise and Physical Activity Recommendations

Regular physical activity has been shown to have numerous health benefits, including reducing the risk of developing stomach cancer. For individuals who have a higher risk of stomach cancer, such as those with a family history of the disease or a history of certain stomach conditions, incorporating exercise into their daily routine can be an important preventive measure. The American Cancer Society recommends that adults engage in at least 150 minutes of moderate-intensity exercise per week, or 75 minutes of vigorous-intensity exercise per week, to reduce their risk of developing cancer.

In addition to reducing the risk of stomach cancer, regular exercise can also help individuals maintain a healthy weight, which is another important factor in cancer prevention. Being overweight or obese has been linked to an increased risk of developing several types of cancer, including stomach cancer. By incorporating regular physical activity into their routine, individuals can help manage their weight and reduce their risk of developing cancer.

For individuals who have a higher risk of stomach cancer, such as those with a family history of the disease or a history of certain stomach conditions, it is important to consult with a healthcare provider before starting any new exercise regimen. It is important to ensure that the exercise program is safe and appropriate for the individual's specific health needs and medical history.

Additionally, individuals may benefit from working with a certified fitness professional to develop a personalized exercise plan that takes into account their individual risk factors for stomach cancer.

Incorporating a variety of different types of exercise into one's routine can help maximize the benefits of physical activity for cancer prevention. Cardiovascular exercise, such as walking, running, or cycling, can help improve heart health and overall fitness levels. Strength training exercises, such as weightlifting or resistance band workouts, can help build muscle mass and improve bone density. Flexibility exercises, such as yoga or Pilates, can help improve range of motion and reduce the risk of injury.

By incorporating a mix of different types of exercise into their routine, individuals can ensure that they are getting a well-rounded workout that can help reduce their risk of developing stomach cancer.

In conclusion, regular physical activity is an important component of a comprehensive strategy for reducing the risk of developing stomach cancer. By following the exercise and physical activity recommendations outlined in this chapter, individuals can take proactive steps to improve their overall health and reduce their risk of developing cancer.

It is important to consult with a healthcare provider and a fitness professional to develop a personalized exercise plan that takes into account individual risk factors and health needs. By making exercise a priority in their daily routine, individuals can take control of their health and reduce their risk of developing stomach cancer.

Stress Management Techniques for Stomach Cancer Prevention

Stress is a common factor in many diseases, including stomach cancer. When we are stressed, our bodies release hormones that can weaken our immune system and make us more susceptible to developing cancer. Therefore, managing stress is crucial for preventing stomach cancer. In this subchapter, we will discuss various techniques that can help you reduce stress and lower your risk of developing stomach cancer.

One effective stress management technique is mindfulness meditation. By focusing on the present moment and practicing deep breathing exercises, you can help calm your mind and reduce stress levels.

Research has shown that mindfulness meditation can also improve immune function, which can help protect against cancer. Incorporating just a few minutes of mindfulness meditation into your daily routine can have a significant impact on your overall health and well-being.

Another helpful technique for managing stress is regular exercise. Physical activity has been shown to release endorphins, which are natural mood lifters that can help reduce stress and anxiety. Exercise also helps improve circulation, boost energy levels, and promote a sense of well-being.

By incorporating regular exercise into your routine, you can reduce your risk of developing stomach cancer and improve your overall health.

In addition to mindfulness meditation and exercise, maintaining a healthy diet can also help reduce stress and lower your risk of stomach cancer. Eating a balanced diet that is rich in fruits, vegetables, whole grains, and lean proteins can provide your body with the nutrients it needs to function properly and combat stress.

Avoiding processed foods, sugary drinks, and excessive caffeine can also help reduce stress levels and improve your overall health.

Lastly, seeking support from friends, family, or a therapist can also be beneficial in managing stress and reducing your risk of developing stomach cancer. Talking about your feelings and concerns with someone you trust can help alleviate stress and provide emotional support. Additionally, joining a support group or seeking professional help can provide you with additional tools and resources for managing stress and improving your mental health. By incorporating these stress management techniques into your daily routine, you can reduce your risk of developing stomach cancer and improve your overall well-being.

How To Prevent Stomach Cancer

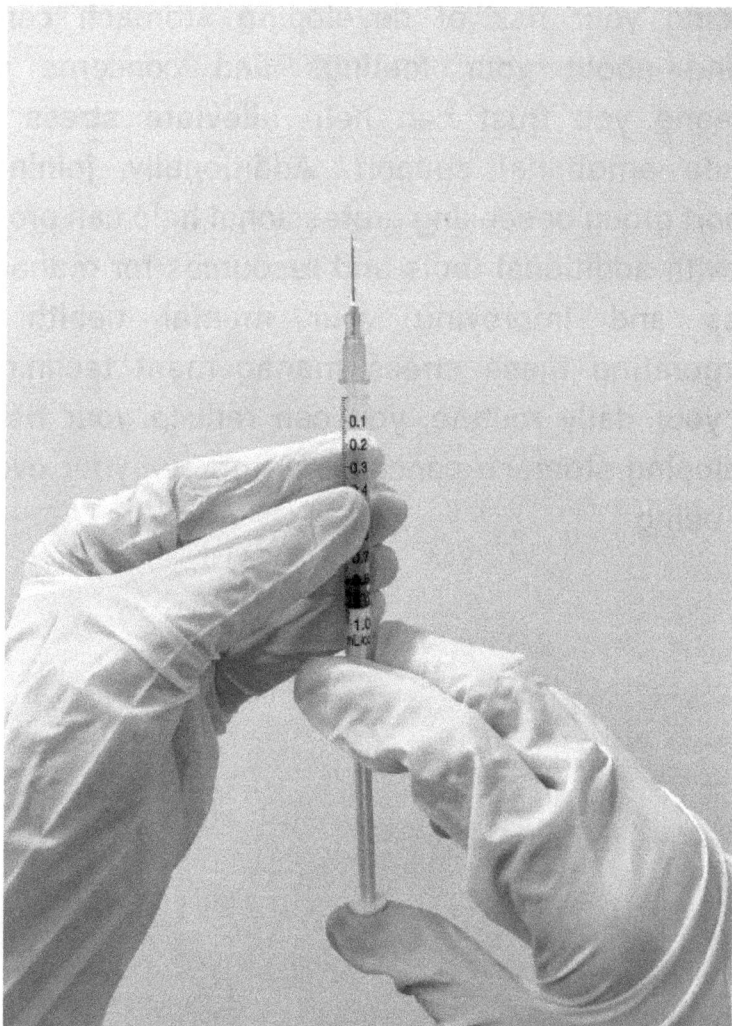

Chapter 5

Medical Interventions for Stomach Cancer Prevention

Vaccines and Medications for Stomach Cancer Prevention

Stomach cancer is a serious and potentially life-threatening disease that affects millions of people worldwide. However, there are steps that can be taken to reduce your risk of developing this type of cancer. One of the most effective ways to prevent stomach cancer is through the use of vaccines and medications.

Vaccines are a powerful tool in the fight against stomach cancer. One such vaccine is the Helicobacter pylori vaccine, which targets the bacteria that is known to cause stomach cancer. By getting vaccinated against this bacteria, you can significantly reduce your risk of developing stomach cancer. It is important to talk to your healthcare provider about whether this vaccine is right for you.

In addition to vaccines, there are also medications that can help prevent stomach cancer. One such medication is proton pump inhibitors, which are commonly used to treat acid reflux and ulcers. By reducing the amount of acid in your stomach, these medications can help prevent the development of stomach cancer.

However, it is important to talk to your doctor before starting any new medication to ensure that it is safe and appropriate for you.

It is important to remember that vaccines and medications are just one piece of the puzzle when it comes to preventing stomach cancer. In addition to these preventive measures, it is also important to maintain a healthy lifestyle. This includes eating a balanced diet, exercising regularly, and avoiding tobacco and excessive alcohol consumption.

By taking a comprehensive approach to your health, you can significantly reduce your risk of developing stomach cancer.

In conclusion, vaccines and medications can play a crucial role in preventing stomach cancer. By getting vaccinated against Helicobacter pylori and taking medications to reduce stomach acid, you can significantly lower your risk of developing this deadly disease.

However, it is important to remember that these preventive measures are just one part of a comprehensive approach to health. By taking care of your body and making healthy choices, you can greatly reduce your risk of stomach cancer.

Surgical Options for High-Risk Individuals

In cases where individuals are considered high-risk for stomach cancer, surgical options may be considered as a preventative measure. These surgical procedures are often recommended for individuals with a strong family history of stomach cancer, a genetic predisposition to the disease, or those who have tested positive for certain cancer-causing gene mutations.

One surgical option for high-risk individuals is a prophylactic gastrectomy, which involves the removal of the entire stomach. This drastic procedure is typically reserved for individuals with a significantly elevated risk of developing stomach cancer, such as those with a family history of the disease or those with a known genetic mutation that increases their risk.

While a prophylactic gastrectomy can greatly reduce the risk of developing stomach cancer, it is important to weigh the risks and benefits of the surgery with a healthcare provider.

Another surgical option for high-risk individuals is a partial gastrectomy, which involves the removal of a portion of the stomach. This procedure may be recommended for individuals with a lower risk of stomach cancer but who still have a heightened risk due to factors such as chronic gastritis or a history of stomach ulcers.

A partial gastrectomy can help reduce the risk of developing stomach cancer while preserving some of the stomach's function.

In addition to surgical options, high-risk individuals may also benefit from regular screenings and surveillance to monitor for early signs of stomach cancer. These screenings may include endoscopic exams, imaging tests, and blood tests to detect potential abnormalities or signs of cancer. By staying vigilant and proactive about monitoring their health, high-risk individuals can take steps to catch stomach cancer in its earliest stages when it is most treatable.

Ultimately, the decision to undergo surgery as a preventative measure for stomach cancer is a deeply personal one that should be made in consultation with a healthcare provider. It is important for high-risk individuals to discuss their options, risks, and benefits with their healthcare team to make an informed decision about their care.

By considering all available options and taking proactive steps to reduce their risk, individuals at high risk for stomach cancer can take control of their health and potentially prevent the development of this deadly disease.

Clinical Trials and Emerging Treatments for Stomach Cancer Prevention

Clinical trials are an essential part of advancing medical knowledge and finding new treatments for various diseases, including stomach cancer. These trials are conducted to test new drugs, therapies, and procedures to determine their effectiveness and safety in treating the disease. For people at risk of stomach cancer, participating in clinical trials can provide access to cutting-edge treatments that may help prevent the development of the disease.

Emerging treatments for stomach cancer prevention are constantly being researched and developed, offering hope for those at risk of the disease. These treatments may include targeted therapies that specifically target cancer cells, immunotherapy that helps the immune system fight cancer, and precision medicine that uses genetic information to tailor treatments to individual patients. By staying informed about the latest research and clinical trials, individuals can take proactive steps to reduce their risk of developing stomach cancer.

One promising approach to stomach cancer prevention is the use of chemoprevention, which involves taking certain medications or natural substances to reduce the risk of developing the disease. These agents may help to suppress the growth of cancer cells, prevent the formation of tumors, or reduce inflammation in the stomach lining.

While more research is needed to fully understand the effectiveness of chemoprevention in stomach cancer prevention, early studies have shown promising results.

In addition to participating in clinical trials and exploring emerging treatments, individuals at risk of stomach cancer can also take steps to reduce their risk through lifestyle changes. Maintaining a healthy diet rich in fruits, vegetables, and whole grains, avoiding smoking and excessive alcohol consumption, and staying physically active can all help to lower the risk of developing stomach cancer. Regular screenings and consultations with healthcare providers can also help to detect any potential issues early and improve outcomes.

Overall, staying informed about clinical trials and emerging treatments for stomach cancer prevention can empower individuals to take control of their health and reduce their risk of developing the disease. By exploring new treatment options, making healthy lifestyle choices, and working closely with healthcare providers, individuals can improve their chances of preventing stomach cancer and leading a healthy, cancer-free life.

How To Prevent Stomach Cancer

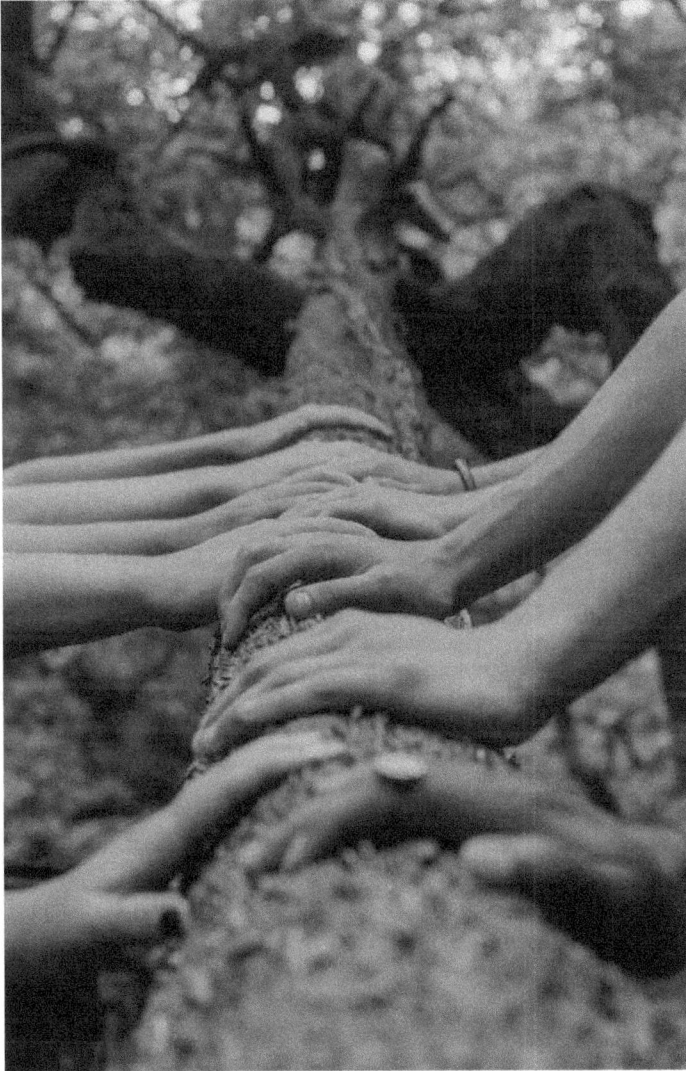

Strategies for Reducing Your Risk

Chapter 6

Support and Resources for Stomach Cancer Prevention

Support Groups for Individuals at Risk of Stomach Cancer

Support groups can be incredibly beneficial for individuals who are at risk of developing stomach cancer. These groups provide a safe and understanding space for individuals to share their experiences, fears, and concerns with others who are facing similar risks.

By joining a support group, individuals can gain valuable knowledge about stomach cancer prevention strategies and receive emotional support from others who truly understand what they are going through.

One of the key benefits of joining a support group for individuals at risk of stomach cancer is the sense of community and camaraderie that can be fostered. Knowing that you are not alone in your journey can be incredibly comforting and empowering. Support groups provide individuals with the opportunity to connect with others who are facing similar challenges and to learn from each other's experiences and insights.

In addition to the emotional support and sense of community that support groups provide, they can also offer practical advice and information on stomach cancer prevention strategies. Members of support groups often share tips, resources, and recommendations for reducing the risk of developing stomach cancer, such as adopting a healthy diet, maintaining a healthy weight, and avoiding smoking and excessive alcohol consumption.

By participating in a support group, individuals can gain valuable knowledge and tools that can help them take proactive steps to protect their health.

Support groups for individuals at risk of stomach cancer can also be a valuable source of motivation and encouragement. When facing a potentially life-threatening illness, it can be easy to feel overwhelmed and discouraged. However, by connecting with others who are in a similar situation, individuals can draw strength and inspiration from their peers.

Support groups provide a platform for individuals to share their successes, milestones, and progress in their stomach cancer prevention journey, which can help motivate others to stay committed to their own health goals.

Overall, support groups for individuals at risk of stomach cancer can be a lifeline for those who are navigating the challenges of living with a heightened risk of developing this disease. By joining a support group, individuals can find emotional support, practical advice, and motivation to take proactive steps to reduce their risk of stomach cancer. These groups offer a sense of community, understanding, and empowerment that can make a significant difference in the lives of those facing this challenging diagnosis.

Counseling and Mental Health Support for Stomach Cancer Prevention

Counseling and mental health support play a crucial role in the prevention of stomach cancer. People who have a higher risk of developing stomach cancer often experience anxiety and stress related to their health condition.

It is important for individuals to seek counseling and mental health support to address these emotional challenges and maintain a positive outlook on their health.

Counseling can provide valuable support and guidance for individuals who are at risk of stomach cancer. A counselor can help patients cope with the emotional and psychological effects of their diagnosis, as well as provide strategies for managing stress and anxiety.

By addressing these mental health concerns, individuals can improve their overall well-being and reduce their risk of developing stomach cancer.

In addition to counseling, mental health support can also be beneficial for individuals who have a family history of stomach cancer. By seeking support from mental health professionals, individuals can better understand their risk factors and take proactive steps to reduce their chances of developing the disease.

This can include lifestyle changes, regular screenings, and other preventive measures that can help individuals stay healthy and reduce their risk of stomach cancer.

Furthermore, counseling and mental health support can also help individuals make informed decisions about their health and treatment options. By working with a counselor or mental health professional, individuals can gain a better understanding of their diagnosis and treatment plan, as well as receive support in making important decisions about their care. This can help individuals feel empowered and in control of their health, which can ultimately lead to better outcomes and a reduced risk of stomach cancer.

Overall, counseling and mental health support are essential components of stomach cancer prevention. By addressing the emotional and psychological aspects of the disease, individuals can improve their overall well-being, reduce their risk of developing stomach cancer, and make informed decisions about their health.

Seeking counseling and mental health support is a proactive step that individuals can take to protect their health and well-being in the face of a high risk of stomach cancer.

Additional Resources for Stomach Cancer Prevention Information

In addition to the valuable information provided in this handbook, there are many other resources available to help you learn more about stomach cancer prevention. These resources can provide you with additional tips, strategies, and support to reduce your risk of developing this disease. By taking advantage of these resources, you can empower yourself to make informed decisions about your health and well-being.

One excellent resource for stomach cancer prevention information is the American Cancer Society. This reputable organization offers a wealth of information on various types of cancer, including stomach cancer.

Their website features articles, fact sheets, and other resources that can help you better understand the risk factors associated with stomach cancer and how to reduce your chances of developing this disease.

Another valuable resource for stomach cancer prevention information is the National Cancer Institute. This government agency is dedicated to researching and preventing cancer, and their website is a treasure trove of information on various types of cancer, including stomach cancer.

You can find information on risk factors, prevention strategies, and screening recommendations that can help you take proactive steps to protect your health.

If you prefer more personalized support, consider reaching out to a local cancer support group. These groups often provide a safe and supportive environment where individuals can share their experiences, ask questions, and receive emotional support.

By connecting with others who have a similar risk of stomach cancer, you can gain valuable insights and practical tips for reducing your risk and staying healthy.

In conclusion, the resources mentioned above are just a few of the many available options for individuals who want to learn more about stomach cancer prevention. By taking the time to explore these resources and educate yourself about the risk factors associated with this disease, you can take proactive steps to reduce your chances of developing stomach cancer.

Remember, knowledge is power, and by arming yourself with information and support, you can take control of your health and well-being.

Creating a Personalized Prevention Plan for Stomach Cancer

Stomach cancer is a serious disease that can affect anyone, but there are steps you can take to reduce your risk. One of the most important things you can do is to create a personalized prevention plan for stomach cancer. By taking proactive steps to protect your health, you can reduce your risk of developing this deadly disease.

The first step in creating a personalized prevention plan for stomach cancer is to assess your risk factors. Factors such as age, gender, family history, and lifestyle choices can all play a role in determining your risk of developing stomach cancer. By understanding your individual risk factors, you can better tailor your prevention plan to suit your needs.

Once you have identified your risk factors, the next step is to make healthy lifestyle choices that can help reduce your risk of stomach cancer.

This includes eating a healthy diet rich in fruits and vegetables, avoiding tobacco products, limiting alcohol consumption, and maintaining a healthy weight. By making these lifestyle changes, you can lower your risk of developing stomach cancer.

In addition to making healthy lifestyle choices, it is also important to undergo regular screenings for stomach cancer. Early detection is key to successful treatment, so be sure to follow your doctor's recommendations for screenings and tests. By catching stomach cancer early, you can increase your chances of successful treatment and survival.

Remember, creating a personalized prevention plan for stomach cancer is an ongoing process. Be sure to regularly assess your risk factors, make healthy lifestyle choices, and follow your doctor's recommendations for screenings. By taking proactive steps to protect your health, you can reduce your risk of developing stomach cancer and live a longer, healthier life.

How To Prevent Stomach Cancer

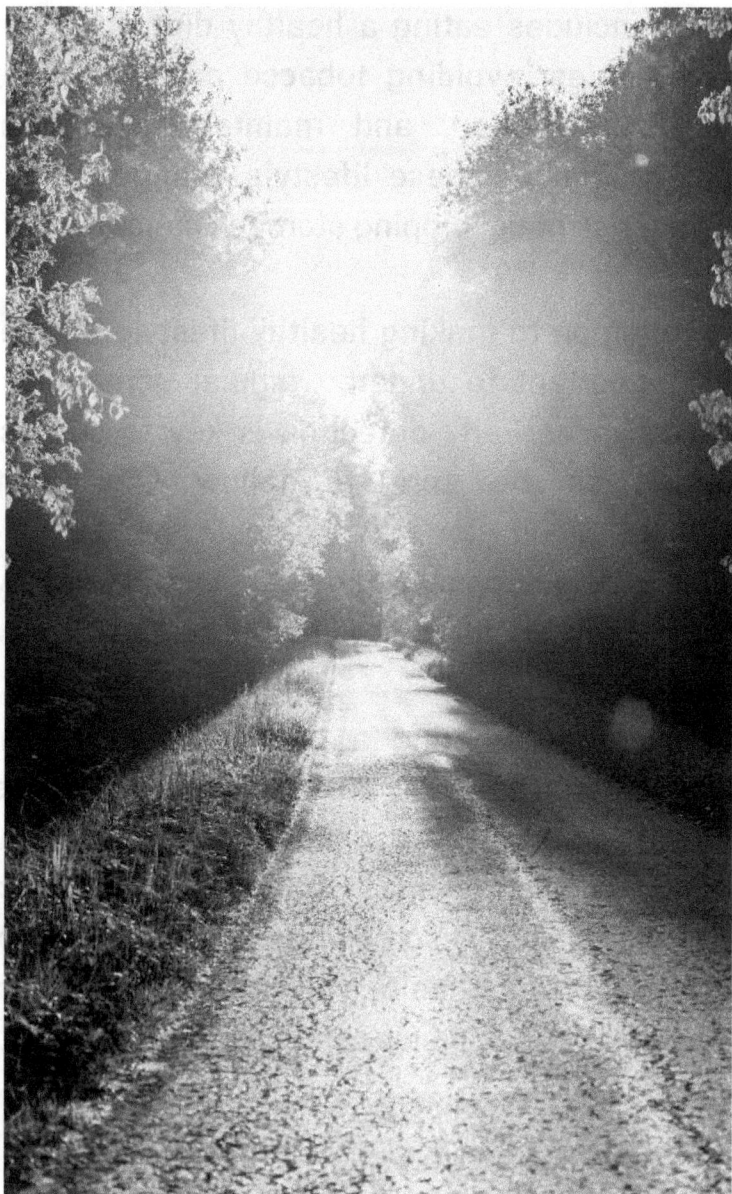

Strategies for Reducing Your Risk

Chapter 7

Moving Forward with Stomach Cancer Prevention

Setting Realistic Goals for Stomach Cancer Risk Reduction

Setting realistic goals for reducing your risk of stomach cancer is an important step in taking control of your health. Understanding the factors that contribute to stomach cancer can help you make informed decisions about your lifestyle and diet. By setting achievable goals, you can take proactive steps to reduce your risk and improve your overall health.

One key goal for stomach cancer risk reduction is maintaining a healthy weight. Obesity has been linked to an increased risk of stomach cancer, so losing weight or maintaining a healthy weight can help lower your risk. Setting a realistic weight loss goal and developing a plan to achieve it, such as increasing physical activity and making healthier food choices, can help you reach your target weight and reduce your risk of stomach cancer.

Another important goal for reducing your risk of stomach cancer is quitting smoking. Smoking has been shown to increase the risk of developing stomach cancer, so quitting smoking is an important step in reducing your risk. Setting a goal to quit smoking and seeking support from healthcare professionals or support groups can help you achieve this goal and improve your overall health.

Eating a healthy diet is also crucial for reducing your risk of stomach cancer. Setting goals to increase your intake of fruits and vegetables, whole grains, and lean proteins, while reducing your intake of processed and high-fat foods, can help lower your risk. Making small changes to your diet over time and setting realistic goals for improvement can help you develop healthier eating habits and reduce your risk of stomach cancer.

Lastly, another important goal for reducing your risk of stomach cancer is getting regular physical activity. Exercise has been shown to reduce the risk of developing certain types of cancer, including stomach cancer.

Setting realistic goals for increasing your physical activity, such as walking for 30 minutes a day or joining a fitness class, can help you incorporate exercise into your daily routine and reduce your risk of stomach cancer.

By setting realistic goals for stomach cancer risk reduction and taking proactive steps to achieve them, you can improve your overall health and reduce your risk of developing this potentially deadly disease.

Monitoring Your Progress and Making Adjustments

Once you have implemented the strategies outlined in this handbook to reduce your risk of stomach cancer, it is important to regularly monitor your progress and make any necessary adjustments to your lifestyle.

Monitoring your progress can help you stay on track and ensure that you are taking the necessary steps to protect your health.

One way to monitor your progress is to keep a journal of your daily habits and activities. This can help you identify any patterns or trends that may be contributing to your risk of stomach cancer. For example, if you notice that you are consuming a lot of processed foods or drinking excessive amounts of alcohol, you may need to make adjustments to your diet and lifestyle.

In addition to keeping a journal, it is also important to regularly visit your healthcare provider for check-ups and screenings. Your healthcare provider can help you track your progress and determine if any additional steps need to be taken to reduce your risk of stomach cancer. They can also provide valuable guidance and support as you work towards a healthier lifestyle.

If you find that certain strategies are not working for you, don't be afraid to make adjustments. Everyone is different, and what works for one person may not work for another. It is important to listen to your body and make changes as needed to reduce your risk of stomach cancer.

By monitoring your progress and making adjustments as necessary, you can take control of your health and reduce your risk of stomach cancer. Remember, prevention is key, and by taking proactive steps to protect yourself, you can increase your chances of living a long and healthy life.

Celebrating Successes and Staying Motivated

In the fight against stomach cancer, it is important to celebrate successes and stay motivated along the way. By acknowledging your accomplishments, big or small, you can boost your morale and continue on the path to reducing your risk of developing this deadly disease.

Whether it be making healthier dietary choices, quitting smoking, or attending regular screenings, every step you take towards prevention is worth recognizing and celebrating.

One way to celebrate your successes is by setting achievable goals and rewarding yourself when you reach them. For example, if you have successfully cut out processed foods from your diet for a month, treat yourself to a relaxing massage or a night out with friends. By acknowledging your hard work and dedication, you can stay motivated to continue making positive changes in your lifestyle to reduce your risk of stomach cancer.

Another way to stay motivated is by surrounding yourself with a support system of friends, family, or a support group who understand your journey and can provide encouragement and motivation when you need it most. By sharing your successes with others, you can celebrate together and keep each other accountable in maintaining healthy habits that reduce your risk of stomach cancer.

It is also important to track your progress and celebrate milestones along the way. Keep a journal or log of your daily activities, such as exercise, diet, and screenings, so you can see how far you have come in your journey towards preventing stomach cancer.

By reflecting on your achievements, you can stay motivated and continue making positive changes to reduce your risk of developing this disease.

Remember, preventing stomach cancer is a long-term commitment that requires dedication and perseverance. By celebrating your successes, setting achievable goals, surrounding yourself with a support system, and tracking your progress, you can stay motivated and focused on reducing your risk of stomach cancer. Keep up the good work, and remember that every positive step you take towards prevention is a reason to celebrate and stay motivated in your journey towards a healthier future.

Continuing Your Stomach Cancer Prevention Journey

As you continue your journey to prevent stomach cancer, it is important to stay proactive and informed about the steps you can take to reduce your risk. One of the most important things you can do is maintain a healthy diet.

How To Prevent Stomach Cancer

Eating a diet rich in fruits, vegetables, whole grains, and lean proteins can help protect against stomach cancer. It is also important to limit your intake of processed foods, red meat, and foods high in salt, as these have been linked to an increased risk of stomach cancer.

Another key aspect of preventing stomach cancer is maintaining a healthy weight. Being overweight or obese can increase your risk of developing stomach cancer, so it is important to stay active and make healthy choices when it comes to your diet. Regular exercise can also help reduce your risk, so be sure to incorporate physical activity into your daily routine.

In addition to diet and exercise, it is important to avoid tobacco and limit your alcohol intake. Smoking and heavy alcohol consumption have both been linked to an increased risk of stomach cancer, so quitting smoking and moderating your alcohol consumption can help reduce your risk. It is also important to stay up to date on your vaccinations, as certain infections such as Helicobacter pylori have been linked to an increased risk of stomach cancer.

Regular screenings and check-ups are also important for preventing stomach cancer. If you have a family history of stomach cancer or other risk factors, talk to your doctor about screening options. Early detection is key to successful treatment, so be sure to stay on top of your health and attend regular check-ups.

By continuing your stomach cancer prevention journey and incorporating these strategies into your daily life, you can reduce your risk and protect your health. Remember, prevention is key, so take control of your health and make choices that will help keep you safe from stomach cancer.

Author Notes & Acknowledgments

First and foremost, I would like to express my deepest gratitude to the people who inspired and supported me throughout the journey of writing this book. This project would not have been possible without their unwavering belief in me and their invaluable contributions.

To my wife, thank you for your constant encouragement and understanding. Your love and support have been my anchor during the challenging times of researching and writing this book. Your belief in my ability to make a difference in people's lives has been my driving force.

I would also like to disclose that this book contains some renewed artificial intelligence-generated content. I really appreciate very recent technological innovation by outstanding scientists and of course our reader's understanding.

Lastly, I want to express my deepest gratitude to the readers of this book. I sincerely hope the strategies and methods outlined within these pages will provide you with the knowledge and tools needed to truly make your life much better. Your commitment to seeking any good solutions and willingness to explore multiple methods is commendable.

Author Bio

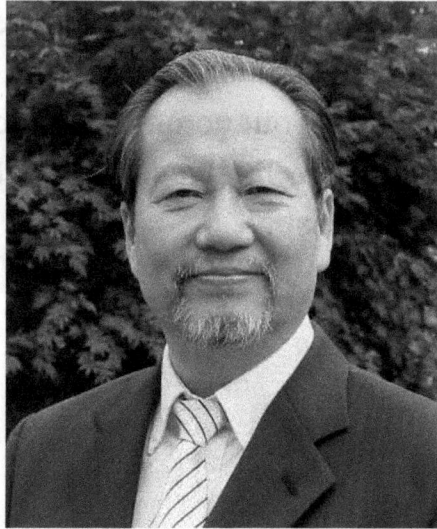

Johnson Wu earned his MD in 1982. With over 40 years of clinical experience, he has worked in hospitals in Zhejiang and Shanghai, China, as well as the Royal Marsden Hospital (part of Imperial College) in London, UK.

Upon the recommendation of Sir Aaron Klug, the president of The Royal Society and a Nobel Prize winner in Chemistry, Dr. Wu was honorably awarded a British Royal Society Fellowship. He has published medical books and articles in seven countries and currently practices medicine in Canada.

www.ingramcontent.com/pod-product-compliance
Lightning Source LLC
Chambersburg PA
CBHW060255030426
42335CB00014B/1716